Table of Contents

Introduction
Special Note Dedication Editorial by Jill Johnson

PHASE- 1..............
Manuel Salazar!

PHASE- 2..............
Navigating through Brain Surgery!

PHASE- 3..............
My Descent into Darkness!

PHASE- 4..............
Friendship!

PHASE- 5..............
Healing!

PHASE- 6..............
Repairing the Holes in my Wings

PHASE- 7..............
Journey into the Awakening by the Light

PHASE- 8..............
Courage!

PHASE- 9..............
He Lived for Me, his path is The WAY!

PHASE- 10..............
Wisdom of the Spirit!

PHASE- 11..............
The Gateway's to my inner Consciousness turned Sanctuary within!

PHASE- 12..............
Freedom, Gratitude!

Tool Box!

Work Sheets...............

Introduction:

Follow the Journey if you can, with a receiving Heart and an Open Mind. In all my experiences, I look for Spirit first. I have used many different names to describe our Creator. I have found throughout this experience, the different names I have used to describe our Creator held different feelings of energy for me. There are many other names that people have used and still use to call the Source of all energy, all Creation. This is a journal account of brain surgery that ended up being a Gateway to an Awakened new consciousness received by the LIGHT. From experiencing the Raw Courage of a young man, as his energy flowed onto me. To a powerful group of people, the Universe aligned me with, to assist in moving me forward in this life.

The inspiration of my books came to me after studying the Spiritual beliefs of many people, past and present today. The experience I had encountered on this Journey I intertwined into a story of studying and having a new relationship with Jesus and following "The Way," as well as the Ancient Essenes that wrote the Dead Sea Scroll, Buddhism, Hindu, Native American Indians, Christianity and many more. And of course, one of the greatest Schools that is always a source of inspiration and complications: the School of Life.

This is a series of events that brought me to an awakening within; a part of me that I thought was new, Awakened by the Light laid sleeping. It brought me to an Authenticity of acknowledging our Creator, on extended levels of awareness. I was blessed with a fresh kindled relationship with the Master Teacher Jesus, Savior to many, that brought a deeper understanding of His living message and how it speaks to me. It is my hope that I can share with you a real-life experience, and how I perceived it and what it had brought to me in my life, from the School of Life.

The Journey that I had taken presented so many gifts, gifts that sat in time. Along with navigating and healing from brain surgery, getting out of my own way, so I could acknowledge their presence. And letting these gifts empower my life, by remembering another piece of who I Am, a gift from the Light
{Our Creator}.

Previous Books by CoCo Saltzgiver: **"The Forgotten Temple"**

SPECIAL NOTE:

To my Mom, your transition from the physical to Spirit left another hole my heart!!!

Mom,

You are in my heart and eventually the sadness will subside. It's a process; I have been here before. Grieving is not an easy process to trust and let it unfold. It's a painful one, yet a necessary one. You have to give the Human experience its due diligence. I will always miss you like Karin, until we cross paths again.

Edgar Cayce said it best:

"Our loved ones don't die;
they just transition through God's other door."

Dedication:

This book is dedicated to Debbie Fitzgerald. Her constant support and reassurance lifted me through some of the toughest, trying, times in my life. Debbie has a very deep way of looking in places where other people never even think to look for answers. She has an innate Wisdom that lays waiting. Debbie's family has always extended their hearts with a welcomed energy of family.

~ Phase 1~

Manuel Salazar!

Where do I begin? I had become a CNA, and I was working for a company that provided service to people in need, due to the fact their needs had changed because of life events, and now need assistance.

I was placed with a young man named Manuel and told, "I think your personality and his will be a good match." I thought, "Ok".

He likes to go out and do things like you. My thoughts were, "ok cool." I asked: "What did he need assistance for?" The answer I got was not what I expected at all.

I was told he was electrocuted on the job, with 115,000 volts not once, but twice and the end result, he lost his arms and legs, hands and feet and burned over 80% of his body. I could not believe it. Not because of what I was told, but because I was wondering how did he live through something like that.

I said, "Ok where do I go and when?" That day changed my life forever. The therapy Manuel needed was extensive as you could imagine.

So, they flew him out to Colorado from Georgia to get the care he needed. Colorado was one of the States that had all the therapy in one place, which could help him heal.

The first day I had the privilege of meeting such a strong soul was a heartfelt day of Honor and deep sadness. He was 22 when his accident happened. Manuel was working at a Rock Quarry pit, when he was asked to unload a Tracker Trailer with equipment on it, for the job.

The Crane that was by him, was supposed to be grounded. It boomed up and hit the power line. 115,000 volts of electricity came down the Crane across the ground and hit Manuel. It surged back on and hit him a second time.

I remember looking at his big beautiful brown eyes and long eyelashes, thinking wow, what a strong Soul he is, and he still smiles.

I assisted him with the shower, getting him dressed and feeding him. Then off to the Doctor's, and then one floor up for Therapy. He told me the Doctors told him he would never walk again. And I said, "And you believed them?"

"Manuel, don't ever let someone tell you what you can and cannot do. People will always try to place their limitations on you."

If it is Doctor's statistics, or just people in general, friends and family. It is usually their fears that they try to limit you to. If you yourself have done everything that you know of and still cannot walk, so be it.

If you find you can, then you walk into the Doctor's office and say, "What do you think of me now." with a big smile on your face.

Watching the pain he would go through exercising his body to get strong, so he could walk on his prosthetics, was inspiring to say the least. His courage was raw, his Spirit strong and always moving forward. It was my first experience of an amazing raw energy of Courage.

I ADMIRE Manuel's endurance; his resilience. He taught me so much that later down the road I would use in making the decision to have the Brain Surgery. Manuel is the face of what a person and their Spirit can endure. He has Dreams of many things he wants to experience in this journey called life. Manuel's attitude shined and his energy expressed was something like this: "BRING IT ON! LET'S DO IT!"

Manuel loved to go to movies. The Bucket List came out. So, off we went. After the show, we sat down and wrote our own bucket list. So I am reading his list when I looked at him and said; "Really, really you want to go skydiving? "He said ya, why not?"

"You're the one who told me I have to try."

Oh, that was me, wasn't it? "My thoughts were, "Ok ya, let's see if they will let you go," all the time thinking they're not going to let him go.

But, like I told him, we have to try, that way we will know; if we don't try we will never know what we can do or what we cannot do.

So, off we went. The whole time I am thinking, "Skydiving, really Manuel."

Well, we got there and I just stood there like a deer in the headlights.

"Initially, I thought to myself, you're seriously going to let him go?" Then I thought, "Ok, let's do it." I was the one scared not him. He was smiling from ear to ear. Me, not so much. We got on the airplane and up we went. You have to go tandem, thank God.

I made sure they strapped him in good. I still could not believe we were doing this. Well, the guy Manuel was tandem with, stood up by the open door of the plane, he looked at me, and I smiled, thinking, "Ok Spirits of the Universe keep him safe." Then the guy flipped out backward's, into a somersault. I looked back at the guy with me and said; "You do that to me I'll slap you." He laughed and said, "I won't."

So, I am looking out the window, no site of Manuel. I just shook my head. I was up, my turn to fly or splat. I thought, "If we live through this one, you're going to get it Buddy Boy." I closed my eyes, and asked God to take care of him.

God: I can't even see him right now. Hold on tight to him.

How can you think anything, but, "WOW look at this kid, with No arms and legs, hands or feet, and we are skydiving."

When we landed, he looked at me with a smile and I said "I take it you had a good time?" He said, *"I never felt so free."*

Now we both know what a bird feels like with its gift of flight.

We also went Snow-Skiing and Water-Skiing. He had no fear. I asked him if he had ever skied before. He said, "You mean with arms and legs?" I said, "Yes with arms and legs."

Manuel replied, "Are you nuts? I would never have done that with arms and legs." I just laughed, thinking wow, "But you will try it without arms and legs."

I felt blessed that he was so willing to experience new challenges in life. Of course, I did not know his limitations or boundaries, and he didn't either. He taught me to not let fear stop you. He was and still is an amazing friend and powerful teacher of life. Manuel is the epitome of what can happen to a person, yet still, go on in life and live it.

Manuel did not allow his accident to define him. He was not Manuel without Arms and Legs; he was Manuel who had different needs now, but still willing to see what life had to offer him. His resilience: astounding.

He is my Hero.

Finishing up our Bucket list, Manuel wanted a family. He now has three beautiful children. He got his family. To watch him interact with his children makes my heart smile.

I wanted to publish a book. My first book was published "The Forgotten Temple". We went on to complete many more dreams on our bucket list.

With our bucket list complete, it's time to start a new one.

A new life for me and a new Bucket list to write. My experience with Manuel, and what he gave to me, helped me make the decision to take a chance at a better life.

My life is so enriched and blessed, with having the people that have come into my life to share it with. A gift was given to me that I recognize, with great gratitude and appreciation.

I found a poem I had written for Manuel one day, as I was watching him workout and try on his new prosthetics to walk.

"Manuel"

You came into my life with a life-changing event, which led to a friendship unbroken. Not time or the twist and turns in life can break that bond we share.

You changed my life for the better. A powerful and rare gift I had received, to engage with such a strong soul.

I felt the Universe and its guiding energy, bring our lives together. Your strength lies in your willingness to continue living life.

With no arms and no legs you know, a part of life most people never would and were still willing to go out into the World and play.

Water-Skiing, and Snow-Skiing, Skydiving and Driving, just to name a few. You are one of the bravest souls I have encountered on this life's journey.

I love to watch you laugh because you still do after all that was taken from you.

You have changed my life forever, and forever I will think of you as the young man who came into my life and was told, he would never walk again.

Manuel, you walked into my life and left your resilience and courage, imprinted on my heart and in my mind for a lifetime.

Amazing and Brave, Gentle and Kind, you
Will always be a powerful force in this life.

A life that made it possible,
to share God with those willing to see the real you
and what you have to offer.
God's strength runs deep through you.

You're amazing, **you are my Hero!**
©2009

As you turn the page, you will see why this beautiful, strong soul has my deepest respect and admiration.

This is what happens when you get hit by 115,000 volts of electricity not once but twice. He still laughs, smiles and dares to dream. He is my hero. One definition of a Hero is: "one who is defined by great Courage, Fortitude, and Noble qualities."

The Spirit Manuel displayed is incredible. I have witnessed all these qualities in Manuel, and his courageous energy rubbed off on me. That is moderately why he is my Hero.

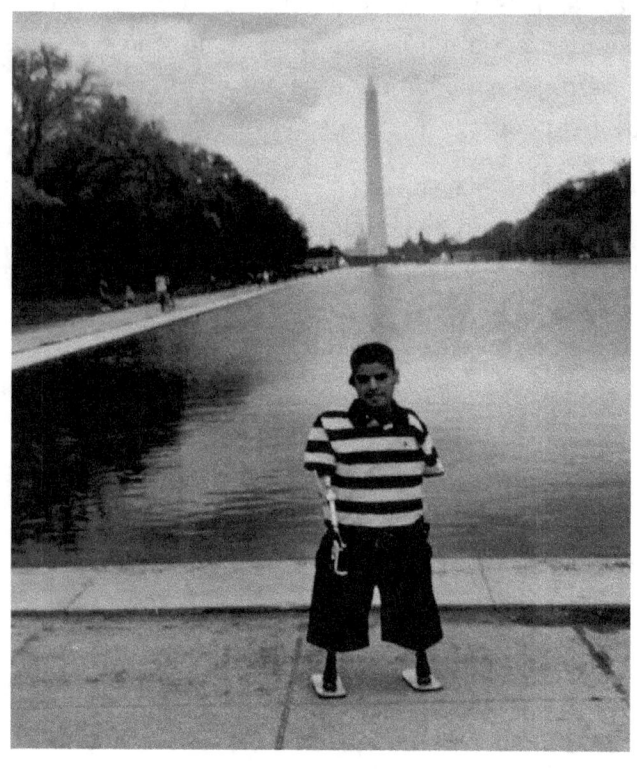

This is Manuel after giving a speech in our Nations Capitol. We are at the Lincoln Reflecting Pool, with the Washington Monument in the background.

~PHASE 2~

"Navigating through Brain Surgery"

It took me a year to make the decision; after all, it was Brain Surgery. It terrified me, but so did the seizures. They were getting worse. The medication was not working; the seizures were coming more frequent. I tried everything that presented itself to me, and I mean everything.

I was not ready to die from a seizure, I just found my Forgotten Temple. I was ready to live again. Live without fear, without pain. I had a whole new life waiting for me. I had found my Inner Temple/turned Sanctuary again, and it was beginning to awaken in places that lay dormant.

As terrifying as it was, there were also gifts that presented themselves in many different ways that I had yet to see and experience. I said yes to the surgery after a year of thinking about it from every angle possible and trying everything possible, not to have to undergo such a Major Surgery.

As the day got closer, I questioned the decision I made. I was terrified. I could still back out, but then there were those seizures that had plagued me since I was thirteen. All those years, of living with the fear of when? How to plan my day and every place I went, just in case. Just in case of a seizure.

I wanted to be free, free to live my life without that fear, that shadow looming over me.

Before the surgery, the Neurosurgeon came in to talk to me to explain a few details. I looked at him and said, "Doctor, I asked God to step inside you and be your hands." He looked at me and said with a grin on his face,

"OK."

"I thought OK, well if nothing else that makes me feel better." For someone who carries the title of a Neurosurgeon, he was a very down to Earth man. That I appreciated tremendously.

On November 17th, 2013, I had a Right Lobectomy that involved removing a portion of the right side of the skull to get to the area of the Brain that was the cause of the seizures.

The first surgery was placing grids on my brain to see where the seizures were coming from. The second Surgery after determining where the seizures were coming from involved, removing an egg size portion of Brain tissue that was damaged due to a Traumatic Brain Injury. All those years of seizures were due to a Brain injury. The swelling from the surgery was painful, or maybe it was how they had my head wrapped so tight that hurt so bad. After all, the Brain itself feels no pain.

As I came out of surgery into the recovering room, my partner Debbie, and my Dear friend / Soul sister, Jackie Sanchez came back and kept my hands down, so I could not rip off the bandage that was wrapped so tight around my head.

It was either that or something to hold my hands, to keep me from ripping off the bandage. I am so blessed to have the people in the life that I have. Throughout the surgery and the healing after, I was never left alone. The whole time I was in the hospital, between my Mom, Debbie, Jackie and Staci, I was never left alone. If Debbie was not sleeping there, Jackie was. My mom made daily visits. I had an amazing support system.

Staci Donahue a friend since High School flew out from Utah to help Deb and myself, not once but twice. Staci could make anyone feel better no matter the situation. She has that energy that lets a person know everything is going to be ok. She stayed the nights Debbie and Jackie couldn't. Staci's sense of humor even right after Brain surgery was welcomed. I should say especially after Brain Surgery.

Amy Orne was always there, either at the Hospital or on the phone seeing if Deb needed something. Whatever way Amy could help she always extended her time. Amy has an amazing gift of humor that I welcome openly in my life and between her and Staci, they had me covered. Amy says just the right thing at the right time, to make life not as serious as it appears. That in itself is a gift.

Ebonni, without asking, always helping out with our animals, or, whatever she could do with the time she had available.

Debbie always had a series of phone calls from my friends in Utah. Nancy O'Toole my spiritual mirror in this Earthly existence. Nadine Tobias she has kept me grounded.

My Uncle Wayne was as close to my dad I could get. My Uncle Wayne and I grew into each other. Our backgrounds could not have been any different. We found common ground. It was not religion, but God that was our common ground. We had great conversation.

I had not shared the surgery with a lot of people. I just wanted to do it and get on in life.

A Nephew I had gotten close to after I told him I was having Brain surgery contacted my brother. I was surprised, he came with his wife. I am so blessed with the people sharing this Journey with me.

The Anesthesiologist before he put me under said, "Go to your Happy Place." I thought, "ok", "can we just do this or I am going to jump off this table and run." Not much time went by, and off to la la land I went.

Debbie told me after I was awake and coherent, that the Anesthesiologist had his Nurse come find her, to tell her as he was putting CoCo under, she was having a conversation with her sister. I just sat there listening to her. My thoughts were, I did go to my Happy Place, and I found my sister. I had not talked to her in 34 years; her life was silenced when it was taken in 1980. I was 20 years old, and she was 24. That same year, it would have been her 25th birthday.

I asked the nurse, so was I over there with her or was she over here with me? The Nurse replied: Oh honey you two met in the middle.

I thought "Good answer and just smiled."

To this day, I do not remember what my sister and I talked about, but I do know she was with me. The Doctors knew nothing about my sister and that her life had been taken by another person's choice he made.

In my room after I was well enough to leave the Recovery room, the friends that came to visit told me I kept telling everyone who came and sat on the end of the bed not to sit there because Karin my sister was sitting there in her yellow summer dress. Yellow was her favorite color. I didn't want everyone to sit on her.

Why have the experience if you can't remember it. Why couldn't I remember what she said? It felt almost cruel. Then it hit me.

She was there, making me feel safe like she always did. Comforting me, through a very frightening time. She came to tell me, to let me know, "I am here sissy, I am here." I always felt safe with Karin and she came once again when I needed her most. Love is the most powerful energy in the Universe. The energy of love is not limited by dimensions or space and time. Love is energy, and energy is all encompassing.

I have always believed, Love finds itself. Whether it is the love of Friends, Family, Animals, the Universe, it will always find its self again and again. Love heals; the energy of love moves people toward their true self within, to the gifts of Spirit within one's self. Not everyone expresses love the same, or believes in what love is. Love never gives up; people do.

I believe love is the energy that holds the World together. When loves not recognized or expressed, everything is in disarray. Nothing feels in balance, all things are in seeming darkness. The light of love that you express will shine bright along your path. It will be a force for moving forward in life. Only you can fill that love within you, and then share it with others. Remember the Greatest Love of all, is learning to love you.

Loving self, is loving the Divine within. There's no ego attached. It's a love of Spirit, with no attachments, no expectations just pure unconditional love. After all, you are an ember of energy from the Divine.

Coming home, Debbie took over the job that the Nurses had performed. She became my Caregiver and was very good at it. Her practice was her Mom, and caring for her through her time of being sick and eventually her Transition from this World to Spirit.

She did an excellent job with her mom, so I knew I was in good hands. It had to have taken its toll on her. After all it was Brain Surgery.

We also had a good fortune, of having Melody Fairbourne, my sister Karin's friend from high school. She had become a Neuro Nurse in Utah and between her and Amber, the Neurosurgeons assistant here in Colorado, Deb and I were covered on all levels.

From the Neurosurgeon and the two Neurologists, everything flowed as it should. One of the Neurologists has a great gift of laughter that in such a serious field brings light to those who hear. The Neuro Nurse always making time to talk and answer my questions, even if I asked her a million times before.

A very special MA, (Medical Assistant) that sees the pain of others and offers a kind word, a smile and a helping hand. All the people that I encountered in the Neurology Department, they always treated me with kindness and respect. I don't think they realize how powerful their words of kindness brought people relief; from the fear they are facing or the fear, they have been living with due to Neurological problems.

Even if it is for one minute or an hour, I smiled and was thankful. I applaud their compassion, their kindness, and patience in helping those, in need. There are many Angels on Earth in many forms.

It did not matter if it was email or a phone call, Melody always got back to us as did Amber without hesitation. Things were good, then the post-surgery Anxiety hit.

~PHASE 3~

"My Descent into Darkness"

What the hell was I thinking?

Descending to hell was exactly what it felt like, there was no light. I kept falling and falling. Was there an end to this descent? Would I see the light again? God, did you forget me? I felt the World drifting away slowly.

The world I knew, the understanding of the life I came to know. Did I make the wrong decision? What did I do to myself? Oh Dear God please, show me you are still there. I felt lost, afraid and alone even though Deb was with me, I felt alone. I did not feel connected to that God Energy and that scared me.

The after Surgery Anxiety was something I never expected. I had no idea anxiety could be so debilitating.

Empty and cold is a better word for what I felt inside. What would the Universe fill me with??? The anticipation of moving through the darkness to see that light again was painstakingly hard. I could see the fear in Debbie's eyes as well. But she always reassured me we would get through it, no matter how much time it took.

Then as it just so happened Amber the Neurosurgeons Assistant, had introduced me to a therapist named Liz, to help me get through some of the dark days that entered my life.

I am so grateful she listened, listened to the Universe whisper that subtle energy asking, to lend a helping hand. In turn, I had been blessed with a powerful person who could see through all the darkness, to help me bring it to the surface, so I could tie together the light again.

The tools she presented to me were powerful enough to get me moving forward in life. The Neurosurgeon helped save my life, Liz helped save my Soul.

The way she could see through me and the pain, it was as if she were peeling off layer by layer of all my pain and fear. That Universal energy was working through her, to help me into the light once more. She did not see it that way, but that's how I saw it.

How else, can that Divine Energy help us, but through other people. People have to listen and then hear where they are being guided to help and who to help. People have to be willing, to be an instrument. When the call from the Universe goes out, those who listen assist.

Several times I had thanked her for showing me that light again and releasing the darkness to do it.

Liz told me; you did it. You wanted to heal, you wanted to move forward and put all this behind you. I just showed you, you could do it. Now that's a good Therapist.

All this was not just the Brain Surgery; the trauma of having Brain Surgery, allowed the opportunity for the other trauma in my life to come out.

Slowly but surely, I climbed grabbing each rock seeing the top of that mountain, it was in site. The anxiety felt like I was being squeezed like a wet rag, trying to get all the water out. I knew this one was going to take time.

The healing from this experience was just going to take time. I got knocked off the top a couple of times, only to find my way back, by the Grace of the Divine and those who felt that gentle nudge to help others.

I have come to learn the virtue of **Patience:** it was a new energy that was foreign to me. Life was fast-lived for me. When you have the kind of energy I have, you are constantly moving just to give that type of energy its due diligence.

I understood Patience on different levels, like watching a flower, waiting to open to the Sun's light.

Watching a Cat stare for hours at what it spotted moving in the grass. That was Patience to me. Once I got it through my thick head, Brain Surgery, it really was Brain Surgery and it is going to take time to heal this one. I learned to settle into it and let it take its long course.

I watched a Caterpillar in its cocoon, transitioning into a Butterfly. Stretching with its new found wings.

What I was becoming aware of was that I had become the Caterpillar once more waiting patiently to transform into a Butterfly and stretch my wings and fly. Like the Butterfly, I had to get my new wings in this cocoon strong before I can fly. The gift of transformation was becoming mine.

I looked forward, never back always forward. Like my therapist said, "CoCo, you had Brain surgery you survived it and its now in the past." Those words alone encouraged me to move forward to the next phase of healing. She would not like this but, she saved me in so many ways. Liz planted the seeds, and I eventually allowed them to grow.
So many people would tell me how strong I was. Friends would call and say; if anyone can do this, you can.

Debbie kept telling me, "You are a strong person CoCo, you can do this."

I would listen and at times think, "Do they know something I don't." I did not feel strong; what I was feeling was downright defeated. My body put limitations on me that needed my kindness. Then it happened. As the days went by I was introduced to a power of energy, it exploded like a ball of light.

Little by little the energy of Light came. It came to fill me up to make me whole again. I had to clean my inner thoughts out. With the new energy, I was becoming aware of my Inner-Consciousness, turning into a new found Sanctuary. I was going through an awakening.

Liz explained to me, the Brain Surgery in its self, was as if it removed not just a piece of my Brain, but a filter. In turn, that allowed all the other experiences that I hide deep down since childhood to come out. Was all that emotional turmoil part of the seizures, besides the Traumatic Brain injury at 13???

I guess I will never know, and that's ok. I don't need to.

The biggest heartache in my life was my sister Karin's Death. I did not know a heart could break so bad. In time, I did not know a heart could heal from being broken so bad. It does take time, and a willingness to do so. As I started healing on deeper levels, another recent heart ache, my mom's passing filled my heart with sadness. **Perhaps, our hearts break to let more light in, and in return let the light out.**

Pieces of my life as a child, and my sister's death came creeping out to be set free. Free, so I could go on to a life filled with Happiness and Love, not a broken heart. That kind of energy is hard to carry, especially in your heart. A person thinks they have healed and released the pain from life's experiences. Then something like this happens and you find there are still fragments of that experience hiding inside waiting and wanting to heal. These fragments stop the light from shining through; it stops you from lighting your Sanctuary within. I don't want to give life to the past. I don't want to feed the past any energy to bring it back to life. I just want to be mindful, and be in the here and now!

I have learned to never put a time limit when you should heal. You heal as time goes on; when you are ready, the Universe will present the right situation the right people to assist in that healing and releasing. Healing is different for everyone. I know I will always miss my sister. I have allowed life to teach me how to live with it. A broken heart now healed. I live with it as a driving force to keep moving forward in life. That's what Karin, my sister, would have wanted.

This experience and what was happening, it was too apparent and it wanted out. Out of me to heal, to let go so I could be free from the past experiences that kept me from moving forward in life.

After all, isn't that what life is all about, evolving Spiritually and growing Mentally? How else do we do that if we are stuck in the past or always living in the future? Living in the here and now and being Mindful of the moment is moving forward to a greater way of life.

Ripping all those bandages off, from the Physical to the Emotional and Mental wounds, was painful. One of my Doctors told me, no one ever tells anyone, how painful healing is. That's probably why most people don't heal, it is a painful process.

Once you get to the other side of all that pain, you've done it. As the physical wounds created from surgery started to heal, the emotional and mental wounds started surfacing, releasing them was excruciating at times. My anxiety was crazy off the charts.

The emotional wounds came flooding out to be healed and released. I was very blessed to have the people that came into my life, to help me through it and to help me move forward again, without all the excess weight. The weight of the emotional pain that I thought at one time I had healed. Their fragments left behind, still waiting to be set free. Alongside memories forgot, now surfacing to be healed.

Karin's death was one of the darkest times in my life. That and the brain Surgery sat side by side. Both experiences were, A Dark Night of the Soul. But she was there, she was with me. Always there with me, oh God I miss her. I miss her simple beauty inside and out and the way she cared for people and life, it just came so naturally to her. It was just, who she was. Maybe that's why her time on Earth was so short.

I began to heal those fragmented pieces. With the help of a good person, who happened to become a Therapist, to facilitate helping people move forward in life. I thank God the hospital had the sense to know, the technology is great, but let's not forget what that technology can do to a human being not just physically, mentally but also emotionally.

The Universe knew her ability to see past where people were afraid to go. Some people hear without knowing, and they are guided to assist others. I thank God that Amber and Liz listened, even if they don't think that's how it happened. I know in my heart of hearts, Amber listened, found Liz and she listened as well. The Universe/Great Spirit calls on all of us to assist, but not everyone listens or hears.

I have been to other therapists, and it seemed like they became a therapist to help themselves with their issues.

Liz was different; she knew how to help people on levels never presented to me before. Did I feel blessed!

The darkness kept peering into my life. Those fragmented memories of a childhood and young adult life, scared by unhealthy emotions, were longing to be free. I kept bringing the darkness to the light that was inside of me. I was surrendering to God and to the Universe.

I kept moving through it, with the Divine by my side, my mom, and Debbie along with Jackie my Soul sister, and many friends. With their prayers and Liz, an amazing and gifted therapist, I kept moving forward.

Karin my sister and Melody's friendship started as high school friends. I smile thinking of the events that led Melody and myself back into each other's lives. Randy and Melody had married; Randy transitioned five years after Karin. Having Melody come back into my life after thirty or more years later was a gift. I felt grateful, blessed and another connection to my sister. The Universe was at work long before all this happened, along with Karin and Randy, I'm sure.

Miracle after Miracle started to occur in my life. That's how I started looking at the World around me. From waking up every day to seeing the Sunshine, the birds in the air and the touch of a comforting hand.

My life had become a miracle to me. I was so blessed in so many ways that I failed to overlook the smallest of miracles life had to offer us, for free. All the miracles were a positive reinforcement of a strong, new foundation that started constructing itself, for me to stand on. The miracles of healing came at different times. Times that I would have liked to be sooner than later.

Divine timing; I let it all unfold in Divine timing. At times, I could not see what was going on around me; I just had to trust the process. Whatever that process was, I know I would come out healthier, stronger and feel a lot safer inside.

I had so much support, reminding me I could do it. The words given to me by so many helped me catch my breath, and breathe again.

So many miracles were abounding in my life. One expression of a miracle As "A Course in Miracles" says, "A miracle is, anytime fear is turned to love that's a miracle." Well, I had plenty of fears that came up to be healed. Through forgiveness, I had released them back to love. I was waking up to a new awareness, an awareness of a life being healed on very deep levels to move forward strong, yet agile. Awakening can be painful, but a necessary process to evolve and ascend in consciousness.

"SO I STOOD"

I looked beyond any place I had dared.

I found power and beauty staring back in an attempt, to rise, with only a Prayer.

Yet how powerful was that prayer?
It changed the intensity of the moment.

The power of immense compassion, filled
An empty heart it embraced.

Once again, a return to a heart filled with love appeared.

A chance to change, a possibility to fulfill the very depths of a life, that was trying to find its way once again through the darkness.

And in return, give that darkness to the Light!

©2014

Witnessing the Miracles around me gave me keen insight into what was right before our eyes. The Seasons were always a sequence of Miracles to me.

Spring:

The Earth takes the first drink of leftover snow turned to water. It brings the seeds that lay waiting for new life. Then the rain comes to replenish the Earths quiet places on the dry ground. Have you ever noticed how beautiful the blue sky is in the Spring? The buds emerge on the trees and bushes. The cycle of life starts again.

Summer:

The Earth blooms new life into existence. The new buds, opening in time to fresh instinctive leafs as they unfold. The flowers open to the warmth of the summer sun. The rivers start flowing with a quick rush, and a longing to immerse itself in the Ocean. The grasses turn green, the days excite with a longer appearance of the Sun. People come out to play. Play in a new Awakened World. Nature is our Creators therapy for the Soul.

Fall:

The Fall air gets cooler, as the leaves start to change. They begin their journey to allow the trees the rest they need, to bud new life again. The grass falls asleep, the air is a little on the lighter, crisper side now. New colors emerge not seen in summer as the leaf's start falling, so the trees can begin their journey into hibernation. The blue sky is now sharp and crisp. Miracles are happening all around us. We just need to be conscious, mindful to acknowledge them.

Winter:

Part of the Earth is in hibernation, preparing for new life. The snow comes and lays in waiting, to give new life its first drink, of the season. The seeds of Fall are laying dormant in Winter's peril. As the snow begins its decent to Mother Earth, she rest. It is as if all life in winter is in a suspended state of contemplation. Contemplating the new life that waits for Spring, arrives.

~ PHASE 4~

"Friendship"

I have been told, I am very rich in relationships. . .

The people that are in my life are there because I believe; we all help each other move forward in life. This is done with support, in helping one another get through life's challenges, along with the lending of a shoulder to cry on or just an ear to listen. These are all very simple acts of love, extended through the light that Friends expand to each other.

Friendship is a place where you can find shelter, from the many impending challenges life throws your way. Friendship is a safe place to give into. Friendship holds the energy that feels safe, to share without judgment, without fear.

Friendship is a special gift of energy that is so welcomed. When the only thing attached to friendship is unconditional love, it can bring you back to the understanding of what it is like to support someone or them in turn support and care about you.

You won't always agree, but you can agree to disagree and still love and accept each other as the sanction of energy, that was brought into your life to share. They love you with all your funny ways and care about you because you give them a reason too. You don't make the energy of love difficult; you just simply love, plain and simple. It's a Love like the Divine. No attachments or a specific outcome waiting. A flow of love, and respect.

True friends know the dark places you have been to and they hold out a hand to say, "Come on I will help you through it. We are in this together."

Friendship is a gift to share on many levels. You will have friends from childhood who may still be your friends into Adulthood. You will meet many friends of all age's, on your life's journey. And in all stages of your life.

Some stay while some move on. The support and caring for one another is a constant flow of energy. Uninterrupted, this energy is always extending the best for that person, on their passage through life.

Most friends help you grow Spiritually. Some are there just to remind you to laugh, and life is just too serious to be taken seriously all the time. Other friends share the same experiences growing up. We can help each other move forward, from what once was a place of pain and fear, to enlighten new views of the experiences we have all encountered.

Friends can reach you on all different levels. Some friends are the ones you know you can tell anything to, and they won't judge you, they listen and pass peaceful thoughts your way with words of kindness and support. These friends are the ones that call you on your stuff, in a kind way of course. Nevertheless, they can tell you in a way that does not compromise yourself or the friendship. It's a call to own your actions.

You know you are blessed when the Universe brings people into your life, in which they become a true friend in Spirit as well as the physical. They are always a secure place to turn, and a comfort from the seeming chaos going on around us.

I will start with the friend I have known the longest and remain in my life today.

1. Nancy O'Toole and I have been friends for 47 years. She is my friend from childhood and a great Spiritual mirror to me in life, now. We seem to go through the same experiences in life, which allows us the opportunity to help each other move forward. Nancy and I share the love of Nature and finding Peace in the presence of the energy of the mountains, and all its inhabitants. Nancy's house growing up was a place of refuge for me, as mine was for her. What I think it really was, it was just being with each other in a crazy time of our lives, as we were growing up. At least we had each other.

2. Sharon: Our friendship started over 42 years ago. We shared many childhood dreams and lessons. We learned a lot together, and a lot apart. We still communicate with each other, throughout time. There will always be a grateful place in my heart for her.

3. Jackie Sanchez: Friends and Soul sisters for 39 years. Jackie is one of the kindest Souls you would ever have the privilege of experiencing life with. Jackie is a shining example with life, no matter what it throws at you that you can still treat the World with a kind and caring heart. As Jackie says, "Choose Love it is everything." Forever and always mug!

4. Staci Donahue: Friends for 39 years. We had lost each other for years, only to find one another as if time never separated us. She is a therapist by nature, and an Artist by choice. She reminds me life can throw you a wall, so walk around it, or climb over it and laugh doing it. Scott, Staci's husband is like a brother to me and a gentle friend. Her sense of humor is inviting.

5. Nadine Tobias: Friends for 38 years. Dean is a consistent reminder of staying grounded. She is a person who no matter what, continues to move forward in life. She has taught me the power of always moving forward and if you have the means to help, always offer assistance to those in need. She is the explanation for, one in a million. Her energy is so easy to be around. She just lets you be. Maynard will always be special between us.

6. Amy Orne: Friends for 29 years. A powerful gift of laughter, always right when you need it most. Amy is right there reminding you life is just too serious to be taken seriously sometimes. She sees the Soul and treats all those in her life with great care and honesty. Mike Orne Amy's husband, told me one day; CoCo you will wake up, and the pain will be gone. It did Mike. The day came, I woke up and the physical pain from the surgery was gone. This is what friends are for. To plant little reminders.

7. Wendy Clark: We have been friends for 27 years. We always walk in and out of our friendship, without missing a beat. Hey, I am here, what ya been doing. Wendy has a gift of vision, to see things that can be, not as they appear to be.

8. The Ulibarri's, have been an extension of family to me for years. Blessed I am, and what a gift to share in life. I will always have a special place in my heart for the love and acceptance they give to me. All the Stars in the sky.

I have met many people in life that have become enduring friends like a local film producer, trying to bring Life and its stories to the screen and sharing in some great conversations. And many who are there to share a piece of time together and move on. I have met new friends and old friend that have become like family to me. From new friends that you share Church with, and a friend that shares the love of the Edgar Cayce material. With each friendship, I feel the importance of sharing this gift of life and the opportunity to help carry each other through life's twists and turns.

Friendship is the Spiritual family you get to choose in this passage we call life. A good example along with the people I have mentioned is the Meditation group Amy and I formed over twenty-four years ago called, "Feed the Light". All the people that have been involved come together to share in each other's growth, and to learn new interest and each person shares at their comfort level.

Our main objective is to Feed the Light in each other and in sharing this it feeds the Light into the World. It is a group of people that want to better ourselves and bring it into the World around them. We help each other evolve.

Pastor Susan of the First Spiritual Science Church of Denver is a welcomed gift of friendship, which was given to me from Spirit. She is a wise, powerful person who has crossed my path of Un-foldment, and has inspired me to trust and believe in my gifts of Spirit.

She is an amazing Mentor and friend. She has guided me with her wise words and actions to believe in myself, and that Spirit within me was indeed guiding me to unfold as I should. As the call comes, I will answer. The First Spiritual Science Church of Denver has become part of my Spiritual Tribe. Sunday morning Services bring a unique perspective for all walks of life. Every Sunday offers something different, the seeds are planted.

I will always have a grateful Heart for her presence and friendship in my life.

~PHASE 5~

"Healing"

I started having dreams that I was not prepared to identify with.

This particular dream was very significant. In the dream, I was shown how all life was connected and flowing through energy. It was the energy of our Creator the energy of our thoughts, and we were all connected. The trees, the animals, and Mankind, all connected with the Earth and throughout the Universe. As I looked at this web of life, it vibrated with a shimmering light that was glowing.

Observing what I thought were little dots spread throughout this massive web, were actually dates. The date I was born. The date my Parents divorced. The ugly date of my sister Karin's Death.

I just stood there looking at this, wondering what this could be. Then I saw the date my Grandma transitioned as well as my Dad and my Aunt Gina.

Then there was the date I found out I had Breast Cancer. The date, we found the guy who killed my sister Karin. It was 29 years after her death, and it took us 3 years and he was made accountable for the choice he made that night. That date shined.

There was also the date of my first book getting published as it was an amazing event in my life. The day, I met Manuel. I did not want to know what those other dates said. The dates that looked like they were in the future. It kind of scared me.

I had to look; the curiosity was getting the best of me. So I did look, but not too far ahead. I saw the date of the Brain Surgery. Then the date I had encountered new teachings, which expanded my consciousness. I thought well that's odd, I studied those along time ago. Why was that date closer to now, this time? Then it came to me. As we grow and evolve with each teaching, it brings us to different levels of understanding. So as we grow, it is like another part of us unfolds, to open up and let additional light out. We should evolve with all people and teachings in our life; the most important evolving process is with self.

I saw another date. I met my Partner Debbie of 20 years. I thought well, that's odd I met Deb a long time ago. Why was that date closer to now, in this time. Then it came to me. We meet each other on different levels as we grow. So as we grow, it is like meeting one another for the fist time again.

I opted out of looking any further, and then I woke up. I sat there trying to piece that dream together when the insight came to me. They were all significant dates that had created a gateway to Life changing experiences. I guess the other dates have yet to be told. I will just keep moving forward, one foot in front of the other.

The dreams kept coming, but this next one, this one brought me peace.

Karin my sister came to me. She was standing there with a dress on and barefoot-like she always liked it. It was dark, but I could see her like it was daytime. I asked her, sissy what did you say to me, what did we talk about during the Brain Surgery?

Karin smiled and said: "I came to be with you so you wouldn't be alone. I knew you were scared. I didn't want you to think you were alone, so I came and sat with you during your surgery."
I asked her how she found me or did I find her? She told me, "We met between the walls of what seemed like darkness to you and light to me." The walls came crashing down to let the sweet abiding radiance come in, so we could share that brief moment in between your time and my no time. That is where we met each other after 34 years."
I smiled and told her how much I missed her and she told me she knew, but I was never alone she was always with me. Karin told me that no one is ever left alone. People feel alone, but they are never alone. It just feels that way...
Then I had a dream I was in a cave, sitting across from Jesus. Everyone around me was talking and I kept saying, "Ssshhhhh are you not listening to this? How can you talk when he's talking?" I sat there with my head in my hands listening to every word, or trying to. Then everyone got up and left, he looked at me and said, "Thank you for coming." I looked at Jesus and said, "Thank you for inviting me." Wow, what a dream. Just to be in his presence of energy.
This is how I want to serve. I want to be Christ like. Those are the steps I strive to walk in.
The dreams kept coming.
I woke up after a dream that seemed so strange like most dreams. I was watching people in India. They were talking about the Cast system they have. The people, in what was considered the lower cast were very sad and frightened. They were looking at the people in the upper cast, not understanding. In my dream, I thought "How strange, when we all breathe the same air."

In another dream, I was sitting in a crowd of people screaming. A bus was driving by really slow. The people on the bus were shouting, and that was getting the crowd going. I turned to my right and Martin Luther King's wife, Cora King was next to me. She was crying and I asked her what was wrong? She told me they have forgotten his message, they have forgotten what he died for. I told her not everyone, I remember. I will always remember.

The dreams started to subside and I was healing now, on different levels. Now it was time to start healing physically.

I had gone through a series of emotional healings and it was time to heal the body. An ancient message of some of the greatest Spiritual teachings, the Human body is a Temple that houses the Divine energy of our Creator. The body is blessed with the job of carrying the Sacred Spirit within. I must treat it as such and allow it to heal.

It is going to take time, every moment of time that is mine to live. I started to live as a conscious being, as I awaken to life around me. Amy and I share a Spiritual connection that we both recognize and honor. It allowed me to come to her in a dream, and tell her I was going to be ok. She said my head was wrapped in what looked like a turban, with all the bandages and I told her I was going to be ok. When she told me that dream, I knew I was going to be ok. I know our connection. I just had to trust the process.

Knowing I had to make this body strong again to continue with the healing. Debbie found a place here in our hometown, called the Aurora Resilience Center. It was set up for people who had faced Trauma mostly for the people who experienced the mass shootings here in Colorado. But, all were welcome. Their receptionist is an amazing Woman name Grace, who greeted every person with respect and dignity. Grace was the heart of the Center.

They offer Yoga as a form of healing, Thai Chi, and NIA along with Mindfulness classes. We had never experienced NIA and what an amazing tool for healing. So every Wednesday, for weeks we went to NIA and continue to experience the healing it offers.

NIA stands for Neuromuscular Integrative Action. As we grew with each class, Deb and I thought of NIA as Now I Am. Now I Am healing, Now I Am releasing. It definitely incorporated itself into all levels of our being for healing. We were blessed with an amazing, connected teacher, Sandy Mighell.

She instructed the class to allow the energy of the moves, to flow through my body at whatever comfort level I was ok with. It allowed you the opportunity to obtain its true healing qualities.

The moves involved in NIA, noticeably helped my body to release trauma for healing. Another tool in my box for healing. The Universe was introducing me to so many different forms that helped in the healing process; at times it was astonishing to see the people that were there to help others heal.

My Therapist suggested it many times until I finally listened and tried Yoga.

It was another art form of healing and releasing trauma. So, Debbie and I started going to yoga. It was and still remains a powerful tool to heal on all levels, not just the physical. I was blessed with another healer, our yoga instructor Lizzy. She brings the Spirit out of yoga into the open, so you can embrace it, in Spirit, Mind, and Body. Meeting Lizzy was like discovering an old friend that our paths crossed again on this Journey. One of many lifetimes shared I am sure. It's such a gift to meet a Soul, and share in how they honor their Spiritual energy. Lizzy gets it. She knows life is a path, that only you yourself can walk. No one can do it for you. People can only offer their experience and the wisdom from those experiences and you allow it to guide you or not.

Debra Thummel, a gifted instrument for Spirit, assured me, "You will get through this CoCo. You have to trust where God has taken you. What you were brought through, so you could move on to your next journey in life."

There are so many listening to the Universe, when it called for those in a position to offer healing, which in turn assist those in need of the healing. I felt truly blessed, with the guidance I had received. I knew it was going to take time. Once you have allowed yourself the process of healing, the wounds that come up, you take the darkness of those wounds and bring them to the light. The process of emotionally healing and allowing the physical body to heal can be a painful one. Let alone the mental piece of having Brain Surgery and anxiety from the trauma of such a surgery and what it released.

I don't think you can put a time on when you should be healed, or when you actually do. Emotionally, there are plenty of fragmented emotions hiding under layers of years ignoring them and the pain that comes along with them. As the Doctor told me, that's probably why a lot of people don't heal; the process is just too painful.

But what is the price of your life, if you don't heal all those wounds. What have they robbed your life of or the people around you? The cost can be enormous, when the energy it takes to keep them at bay, it is so apparently immense. To keep deflecting those painful experiences on to people around them by not healing them, will eventually take its toll on the people they love and the ones that love them.

"I STAND READY TO AWAKEN"

Oh, Creator, I stand ready to awaken in my truest form.

I know not where to go, or where to look.
I know not my life and its boundaries.
Creator, do you have a Divine plan waiting for us all? Is it all in the power of your truly beautiful name?
Is it in the power of Prayer?
I can feel your energy, your peace, your contentment.

I stand ready to Awaken, ready to emerge forth as a powerful light being.

I am Spirit, and my Spirit is intensifying to a new expression of life on Earth.

©2013

~PHASE 6~
"Repairing the holes in my Wings"

Another heart ache, my mom's passing, filled my heart with sadness. My mom told me before she died, "CoCo I know what you are doing. You're repairing the holes in your wings." Mom, you left this World and now I have another hole to heal and repair. Healing I have learned, is a huge part of life. Death is a very hard teacher. My mom and I had gotten very close in the last years of her life. Her passing was so unexpected.

My heart is sad, very sad. My mom was intelligent, funny and very gifted in Spirit. I will miss our walks together every morning for three miles a day. At 83, she was still walking 3 miles with me. We would stop at one of the ponds where she lived, and sit and pray together. Her resilient Spirit was an amazing legacy to the life she had experienced. A tough life lived not an easy one at all. She taught me well. I look back and see how much I learned about the things I have come to enjoy, and they were given to me from my mom. The solace I have found in her transitioning is that she is with my sister Karin. Karin was the oldest. That had to have been an amazing reunion when they saw each other on the other side. My mom had told her neighbor she missed her daughter. "Well mom you don't have to miss her anymore. Now I miss both of you. I look forward to that day of being reunited with both of you again."

"I love you mom, and I miss you on many levels of the physical life I shared with you. Mom, you are in my heart and eventually the sadness will subside. It's a process, I have been here before. Grieving is not an easy process to trust and let it unfold. It's a painful one, yet a necessary one. You have to give the Human experience its due diligence. I will always miss you like Karin, until we cross paths again."

"So until then mom, I will finish repairing the holes in my wings. I will continue to grow and evolve my Spirit. I will listen for you in the sounds of the birds singing, the squirrels chattering and the Blue Heron flying by in the sky. I will walk with you in the Mountains and throughout my life."

~PHASE 7~

"Journey into the Awakening by the Light"

Having found myself within, an awakening of Authenticity started to construct itself in me, at a level I found easily comfortable. The light came and that is when the fear started to break away.

The new life was growing inside of me, and it started taking on deep roots for a very strong foundation, once I got past the hollowness. It was a new Sanctuary in the making, what and when could I start living in this new self.

Feeling empty at times, wondering what would the Universe fill this empty heart with, kept nudging me to listen. The anticipation of moving through the darkness to bring it to the light again was painstakingly hard. I knew at times the Universe was giving me just what I needed at the time I needed it, to make myself shine.

Friends and family always reassured me I would get through the healing no matter how much time it took. I thanked God for these people being by my side, and it was then, I felt that familiar energy of LOVE enter my Heart. Throughout this whole experience, it filled me with Unconditional Love.

The most powerful energy in the Universe, **LOVE**. The energy of, Unconditional Love was filling my Consciousness within.

My thoughts racing, is there going to be room for anything else? This energy of Love was unreserved ahead of my understanding. It felt as if Heaven had opened its doors and a piece fell out into me.

Little by little the gifts came, and I felt the emptiness give way to an energy that brought in the beginning of an awakening to new life within. I had worked so hard to clean my consciousness out, and now I was filling all that space with new life. I had gone on a Journey of wanting to make this life better; into the descent of darkness, that many have called "A Dark Night of the Soul".

I have experienced it a few times before and had the insight to find it was the rebirth of the light of a new life. I just had to get through it and try my hardest to trust the process.

Between the thoughts, it all came crashing down. Places of darkness had turned into places of sweet unbinding light. It was as if the Brain Surgery had become a gateway to an Ancient Spiritual Realm of recognition.

This energy occupied a place inside of me, to bring into being, a new breath of life within me. It took on an awareness all its own. It was as if a birth of new light was just beginning to peek through my Spirit, I was experiencing an Awakening. I fell into a World of unpredictable emotion. I waited and watched as the light found its way inside of me. "Trust the process," I kept telling myself, "trust the process…"

"Awakening"

In the beginning there was light, there was always light.

The Darkness was the shadow of the light that fell upon those who had fallen asleep to who they are.

They started to awaken and recognize their true self, as the light. The darkness dispelled into the oneness with the light.
The shadow was gone and the Soul set free.

Free to blend, free to just be and free to live life Awakened and in peace!

©2014

The energy reached levels of a deep awareness, **Gratitude**. Once again, my consciousness was now overflowing with Gratitude.

An origin so forthright, that it brought me to an understanding of self. Having never experienced this feeling or had this kind of awareness, it was in anticipation of a chance I took, to have a new life. It came into sight starting from inside, working its way to the outer core of my energy.

The new life I wanted…A life without seizures and without fear was emerging.

Seeing the persistence Liz had, in helping me move forward, filled my consciousness with **Determination**. An added energy had found its place inside of me. I was being filled new again. Was there room for more I thought? Or was all this just Unconditional Love, bundled up into one immense, beautiful, powerful, force with many facets to it.

My Spirit was being filled again; it was healing the darkness inside. Liz may have thought it was just me, but I knew as God did, Liz was giving me the exact tools I needed to bring the light back in. Her gifts are many and I know she can help others that are fighting their way back to the light. Whether it's from Brain Surgery or Seizures or just life itself.

So many people would tell me how strong I was. Friends would call and say "If anyone can do this you can." Debbie kept telling me," You are a strong person CoCo, you can do this." I would listen and at times think "Do they know something I don't." I did not feel strong, what I was feeling was downright defeated at times.

Then it happened. As the days went by, I was introduced to a power of energy that exploded like a ball of vibrating light.

Strength, it started expanding from my head to my toes and everywhere in between. I heard a whisper of words telling me, "This was always in you, all the energy that is awakening to a new life." It was just waiting, waiting for you to let go of the fear of who you truly are. I contemplated, who I truly am, "Ok show me Great Spirit who I TRULY AM." I thought I knew.

Little by little the energy came. It came to fill me up to make me whole again. The gifts kept opening slowly, and one by one they were awakening.

As this energy of Strength started to grow, I became much more accustomed to it. I did remember feeling this throughout my life. This was a bit different though. This time the fear of being strong, was no longer attached to the manifestation of its energy and what it meant. Strong, yes I am strong, but not in the way so many people see me as.

My strength began in childhood, then as a teenager a young adult and now in my fifties. It was as if the Child of the Universe that I am, that we all are, was awakening to my true Authentic self, and accepting it without fear. The ego was falling away.

The key to recognizing the difference between living in the Ego or Spirit was acknowledging living a life without fear. Fear is Ego based. I was beginning to release the fear of a conditioned life and accepting who I am. Knowing it, and believing in it, allowed me to no longer fear the Past. What a layer of energy to release, and replace the fear that once plagued my life with the energy of Strength. It is a Strength of Spirit, a gentle all-encompassing strength.

I had become strong: strong to be the person I am with self-acceptance and awareness, that's my Strength. It is a strength that comes not from this world but, from Spirit. It is within and if it happens to spill over and onto the outer part of my Energy, I welcome it.

Little by little the energy came. It came to fill me up to make me whole again. I had cleaned my conscious thoughts with the things I could see, and trusted the Light to clean out the rest of what I could not perceive. Birth, is always painful and at times, this new birth felt like a magical awakening, bringing me forth to a steadfast beginning. It was happening to me, so I could extend life outward to the World and all its inhabitants around me.

I knew if it was happening to me on this level, it was happening to everyone to some degree. It was the Universe bringing new energy to the Earth. Whether they felt it or acknowledged it, these were the gifts waiting for all. The gift of becoming free from the man-made emotions left over from pain.

It was a quite Awakening, gently pushing Mankind forward. Knowing now at this time, the journey had its own intent. The intention of this new energy would find its way into people's lives. It just happened to find me through Brain Surgery.

Even though my experience I thought started with the Brain Surgery, it had been with me throughout my whole life. Nudging me, reminding me, and always beckoning me in everyday experiences of life. The Brain Surgery was a huge push to allow the Light in, without having to get out of my own way, for the Universe was doing it for me.

I could have said no to all the changes taking place, but why? When you recognize the gifts in such a frightening experience, you bless them, hold on to them and move one foot forward. Just keep moving one foot forward.

The power of the Universe is changing; it is time to bring in a rewarding and renewed life. It will need little words to describe its vibration once you experience this new awareness. It can stand on its own.

To obtain a river of light, wrapped up in a never-ending always evolving Universe and to be able to find it within you, is powerful. And to hold onto it is a captured moment in what we call time.

For me, the Light was waiting to get out. Sharing in its liberation, it waited to embrace a Soul longing to find its way back. Back to a place of unshakable tenderness and compassion. It is a Sanctuary of a love, a love that is Divine in nature. So powerful, it speaks of a solemn Journey of awareness and service. Service in itself is a gift, to those who cross your path, and that gives you the gift of remembering.

Remembering your oneness, your connectedness and your ability to forge ahead despite the adversity you have faced or are facing. The Wisdom to know you, on levels not expressed before. Love and an Ancient feeling of Togetherness will give you the opportunity to explore the unexplored. You are free to accept these gifts that are given to all. If you choose to accept them, pass it on to those you meet. These gifts were never meant to be held in place, but to give to those you walk in everyday life with. I had watched Courage express itself, through other people and Animals and now it was emerging in me with a new appearance.

Looking back on my life, I had courageous moments throughout it. As told I had a young man Manuel, share his courage with me, yet I never really held on to it or acknowledged it was something I had. Now, I was feeling it inside and allowing it to flow into and onto my outer presence.

This was a surreal awareness, and it was as if the chains of thought that no longer represented or served the Spirit of my inner consciousness were being replaced with the gifts of thought that our Creator gave to us all. Thoughts and feelings of a life lived in Truth and Peace, a life lived from Spirit first. Away from fear and mankind's limitations of life and how Society dictates how one is supposed to live it, away from life lived in Ego.

The chains were falling off but the biggest one had a ball on the end of it. I like to think of my Neurosurgeon as a gift, a gift that presented itself in perfect timing with the Universe. He did unlock that ball and chain from my leg I had been dragging around since I was 13, the chain of seizures from a Traumatic Brain Injury. I will forever be grateful for him. I was being offered the gift of freedom, freedom from all that was placed upon me from other people's fears, and their beliefs about life. Along with the freedom from self- imposed thoughts that enforce the fears. Fears that do not serve my higher good, and those around me.

The new life that has presented its self to me is one that I can open my Heart and Mind, to be in Harmony with all life. We are all one, and I was ready to take my place in God's one big family.

As my persistence continued in allowing time to heal my body, which in turn, continuously healed my mind and my Emotions, it brought me to an Awakening. My Spirit knew that the Genius of it all, this had all been orchestrated from the beginning of my time, here on Earth.

Everything I had gone through, was going through, would go through, it was all happening so I could have the chance to have a better life and a chance to evolve my Soul. The light would always penetrate the darkness that we stand in and offer up.

The energy that came in, it was as if it represented a life frozen, a life lived with fear always looming behind, not knowing something like this ever existed. Then it shattered into a million tiny pieces. Pieces that represented a fragmented life, torn apart by emotions. Fear that released its own negative impacts on a life meant to excel, to shine. It was the freedom to be me, and when I say me, I mean the freedom to express my deepest authentic knowing, of the Divine within me.

The true Spirit of my energy, that energy that runs through all life, all Creation had found its way back inside of me. The energy of the Earth, the Animals, the Ocean and the Mountains, our Creator had found a way to enter into my energy, on a level that thrust me forward. Forward, to a new and powerful Authentic Awakening, an awakening through Brain Surgery, by the Light.

It was an energy so encompassing, it filled my very existence of the Human Life I was living. It was a new way of living life, to share and give to others. The energy was a reminder that we are Co-Creators on this Journey we call life. We Co-Create, through our thoughts, our actions and our spoken word. The amazement of such energy filled me, with the beauty of a life being recreated, through the powerful presence of our Creator. This energy whispered of an ancient knowledge, it was time to remember. **Within us all, is the Divine Wisdom that lays waiting.**

Waiting to burst forth and embrace the self that's willing and ready to accept this energy, bound forth on a new level of consciousness. The song will be sung for all to hear. The air will delight in each breath taken.

The wind will gently move through the trees as if they were dancing. The tall grasses will sway in harmony, as this new energy is awakened. The animals will feel the same vibration that accompanies the changes. They will begin their song with chatter, then a cry from the sky and a powerful howl from the mountains below. All forms of life are being prepared. The intention is to flow into a harmonious union of creation. A transport, into awareness, like no other.

It is a powerful new beginning unto its self. It will end joyfully. The energy is a courageous Authentic Awakening to those who allow it. It will be like waking from a dream so real, so beautiful you have to share it. What you will share, is the Light of the Divine. It is blissful, peaceful, a congruent of possibilities. As we unite ourselves with the Divine, and the power of this new energy it will remind us, that life can be very forgiving. Give life a chance, and it can right that which seems wrong. The World as we know it is changing. It is changing for the good of the Whole.

It will be a reckoning of separation, to the awareness that all life is one. The power of the Authentic self is constructed on levels beyond the senses. This World seems blind to the Spirit of Life. As we grow and evolve our Souls, we can begin to see the energy of Spirit in all Creation. This energy connects all life together as one. The only separation is in the minds and Hearts of those that fear change, fear the unknowing and fear themselves. Fearing yourself you will involuntarily fear others. Being Authentic to self is a critical decision on the part of the person trying to evolve their Soul to a new level of understanding and awareness. Once this understanding is applied and the awareness embraced, the old fears will give way to a comfort of new life.

The newly Awakened consciousness will rise within you. It is awareness, a remembrance of life meant to be lived. It is the life of Spirit that knows all paths and lives it as a gift of recognition to the Divine within. We are all the authentic embodiments, of the Divine within us and all around us. All Creation embraces the Divine Energy because all energy was created from the Divine.

There is a constant internal knowing that we are all the living, breathing Temples of the Divine Life Force. The Spirit of our Creator within us is always reaching outwardly, to connect, to share and give back that which has been given to us. Over the years of living life, the experiences are all meant to be shared. We are all being called, to bring ourselves and those around us to the Divine Spirit within. It is a constant strand of energy that vibrates through the physical life, calling us back to our true selves. Like the never-ending flow of the Universe, it is constantly expanding and breathing new awareness out of the space that surrounds it.

Given the precise circumstances at times without you even knowing it, you can begin to see the light as you grow and evolve your Soul. It will present itself to you in many forms like the gentle whisper of the wind. It is a spoken set of words, that change your insight, your perception.

An event you experience personally or a world event that has taken place, or an illness. It may be the transition of a loved one. It may be as simple as the words in a song or it could be the laughter and joy you share with others. There are many gateways that can awaken a person to change. That change can bring the needed tools to let go of the old and that which no longer allows you to move forward in life.

You can awaken to a new awareness simply through observing Nature. The Universe is unlimited, in how it can achieve directing one to awaken to their true selves, which will assist in evolving one's Soul. People limit themselves to what they can do and achieve in life. I believe the biggest factor is fear. Fear of the unknown the known and a World at times that does not lend one a lot of hope. It is fear that the Ego loves to keep us in.

Spirit is love, and love moves us forward.

"Today I Rise"

Today I Rise to the swelling Spirit within me.

I Rise above the artificial noise of this World, to hear Spirit inside me. I Rise to the calling of life, as it beckons me to move forward.
It's time to live, it's time to Rise.

I Rise to a powerful existence of love, unfolding into a prevailing continuation of awareness.

I Rise to meet the call, I Rise!!!

©2015

~Phase 8~

COURAGE

To experience **Courage** is a gift that unfolds in its own time.

Throughout the healing process, Courage started awakening inside of me. It wasn't a Courage of I did it. More like, I did that zip line across a canyon feeling it gives you. It was a feeling of no matter how frightening or feeling like crap you felt that day; just keep moving forward one foot in front of the other. Just keep moving forward. That took courage. I witnessed this courage in a young man, hit by 115,000 volts of electricity twice. (Manuel)

Courage is an energy felt on so many different levels.

Courage to speak up, when no-one else does. Courage to go against the mainstream of society, when you know in your heart it's not right.

To try new experiences in life, and to really put yourself out there that takes courage. The Courage that presents itself when life knocks you down is a whole new Spirit of Courage. You find it inside yourself. It's a place that pushes you forward. Whispers, keep moving don't stop. No matter how bad you want to, don't stop. Get out of bed, get dressed put your shoes on and start moving. One foot forward just keep moving.

This kind of Courage is you not being defined by the life experiences that knock you down. It's the Courage that rallies you within, to start living life again. I let this feeling grow inside me, every time I felt the fear or non-understanding start to pull me back down.

I learned this type of Courage could take my experiences, and change my life for the better. Instead of allowing it to beat you into the ground, you can rise within yourself and keep moving and keep living life.

Courage can allow you to open your heart to the World, so you can experience life on many different levels that it presents to you. Sure, you can curl up and close your heart off. How does that serve you and the World you live in? Sometimes just getting up one more day and moving forward is courageous in itself. Courage for those who seek it even in the face of fear, these people rise up and move forward. Regardless of life's experiences that knocked them down.

They move away from that experience that knocked them down, towards a great light that shines as a Beacon in the Darkness.

Courage moves one forward to Compassion for oneself and in turn, for Mankind and the Earth with all its inhabitants.

Courage is the Spirit saying yes when the Ego says no, I can't.

~PHASE 9~

He Lived for Me, his path is The WAY!

Jesus Lived for Me. You always hear Jesus died for your sins. I came to the awareness that Jesus lived for me. Now I wanted to live for what he taught. Jesus' teachings are so simple. His spirituality is amazing. Jesus' teachings were meant to be Universal.

"Love one another as I have loved you. Judge not lest thee be judged." So simple when saying it, seemingly hard acting it out in life and applying it. Effortlessly spoken words, "Though shall not Judge lest thee be judged, Love one another as I have loved you."

How could these words get so misconstrued? Jesus showed me a way I could walk in this life. He gave us the tools we need, to save ourselves from ourselves. We have to do the work on our own self. Our Soul and this life are our responsibility to heal and evolve our Spirit.

Bring forth all that is within you, it can save you. Keeping all the darkness that is within you, can rob you of your life, and all the happiness that could be yours.

They brutally tortured and crucified Jesus, because of the messages He brought to this World. So did He die for me, if you choose to look at it in those terms, He did die to bring in his teachings, his message to show The Way, to save ourselves from ourselves. Simple is His message and we make it so hard. Jesus' words are one with Spirit. He came to set us free. Free, from ourselves.

I choose to look at Jesus as a very Spiritual being. He is the presence of the Divine Energy of life. Jesus was the man, the Christ energy was the consciousness he brought to the Earth. God has many faces on Earth. These Faces represent life here on Earth in all forms, to help all his creation find that path inside, which can lead them on their Journey back to the light. Jesus' words can be practiced in any Faith or Teaching, that's the Universal Being Jesus is. "Love one another as I have loved you. Judge not lest thee be judged." That was his Way. I want to be a follower of his Way. In the times of his teaching it was called the Way, and believers were referred to as "Followers of the Way." (Book of Acts from the Bible)

These are Powerful words that can strip away the harm that Mankind places on one another, or what we place on ourselves. If these words are put into practice and not just spoken, they can create a path of least resistance to life.

Jesus gave us the tools to be our own Savior, and heal ourselves. What do most people need to be saved from? Themselves, of course. As we heal ourselves, in turn, it helps heal the World. Religious or non-religious, Spiritual or not, Jesus' words can be incorporated into a person's everyday life.

I always wondered when Jesus said: "My Father's house has many Mansions in it." (John 14:2.) What that saying could possibly mean. I really took note. As I began to Meditate on this, what came to me made sense to me. What does a Mansion have, but many rooms? There are rooms upstairs, downstairs, and on the main floor of a mansion. God is the Mansion and in God are many Levels. The rooms are all levels of conscious understanding. All paths lead back to the Source {God}.

That spoke to me. With the purpose of the Divine being unlimited in consciousness, it brought me to the awareness that all His Children can come back home in whatever level of consciousness they have obtained.

There are many rooms, so people can always grow in their awareness of God. God is unlimited. The only thing that limits our Creator is our own Perception or knowledge of the Divine.

Jesus was a Master Teacher on Earth, which showed us a powerful path that we could walk to return to our true selves.

Jesus is a brother, a friend and a Savior too many. Jesus is a light at the end of that long road to home. Some of my favorite teachings are Jesus and Buddha.

They both taught Awareness and or Enlightenment. Both believed and practice one of the greatest of teachings, "Thou Shall not Judge, lest thee be judged." (Jesus.)

"Do not be the judge of people" do not make assumptions about others. A person is destroyed by holding judgment about others." (Buddha.)

I stand, and before me is the power of choice. It is the power to articulate, a new and opulent life. Our Master Brother Jesus created a new way of life thousands of years ago. A life lived in Love and Peace through non- judging and loving one another. I believe this is how He overcame this World. He overcame an Ego driven World, by rising above it, to live his life in Spirit. What is Spirit's most powerful energy consists of? Love of course.

I was reading a Book called Jesus before Christianity by Albert Nolan.

Staring at the name JESUS, written in big letters I started thinking, how Jesus name in his written language of Aramaic is Yeshua. Then the insight came to me.

The name Jesus, in his written language of:
Aramaic was Yeshua.
It got changed to Jesus, in the Greek language.
In Spanish it's Jesus
The J sounds like an H in English.
So if you spell it how it sounds with an H, Which is Hesus,
staring at it and meditating on it, it hit me.
Hesus, "HE'S US"

"Jesus is us".

That Awareness brought about, through Meditation an accepted wisdom about Jesus. These are just a few pronunciations of his name. Throughout all the different languages there is still the same energy.

Still the same person with the same message, just many different ways to say his name...

Jesus said "I AM The Way, the Truth and the Life." He embodied the I AM presence. What he taught as the Way, is Love one another as I have loved you, Judge not lest thee be judged. He walked his talk.

Living this in everyday life, you will find TRUTH and that truth will lead you to a new life.

A LIFE, in the consciousness that Jesus taught us all and shared with all. He showed us the Way the Truth and the LIFE and that is the path he walked and presented to us the opportunity that we to could walk it.

His consciousness can be our consciousness. Living his message is living Christ-like and that I believe is the key to obtaining his consciousness and overcoming this World.

"Be in this World, but not of it." (John 17:14-15)

Day to day living can be hard enough. Being Mindful of that moment to moment and what you are putting out to the World, is an accomplishment in itself. If we practice living a life, of loving one another and Judge not lest thee be Judged, our whole lives and everything around us will change. Be in this World but know, everything and everybody is temporary. So don't make this world apart of you. Just be and experience it.

This poem was inspired by a meditation on Jesus life!

I come to you in so many ways.
In the crisp Autumn morning
In the cool days of Spring
I reach past all barriers and give you my love.
I lift your energy in the morning light
I bring to you an embrace at the closing of the night I am always with you and all around you
My light is your light
I whisper in your ear from an ancient sound of love

I will always be with you on your Journey in life until you return home with me!

2017©

Jesus and I have become good friends. He is like a brother to me and at times a Savior. Jesus can be a Savior if you need to be saved from something; usually it is from our selves. His living words saved me many times, as I have gotten out of my own way and let His words speak to me. I have learned how blessed I am, to have the awareness of consciousness and to share it. I want to be **Christ Like and walk The Way**, as I live out my life, on this beautiful gift, that we call Mother Earth. Jesus hurt no one. He loved everyone and judged no one. "I to aspire to be **Christ Like**."

Jesus said; "That man shall not live by bread alone, but by every word of God." (Matthew 4:1-11).

Thinking and meditating once again on this saying, brought me to the understanding that man cannot survive by just feeding the Physical. We also have to do the work and Feed the Spirit. You have to do the work for yourself.

Taking care and feeding your Soul is an everyday job. Bring Prayer into your life. Read Spiritual sayings, and or Spiritual books. Meditation, Mindfulness. Walk and have a conversation with the Divine. Whatever speaks to your Heart, give that gift to yourself.

Practicing Yoga, NIA, hiking, for example: there are so many ways to feed your Spirit. Service to others in many forms and writing, just to name a few.

These are just some ways to connect back to God. What in your life connects you back to the source? What do you feed your Spirit?

However you believe in our Creator, start by acknowledging your Spirit through the spoken word. The Spoken Word is powerful. There are many times I have talked aloud to God, and listening to the answer has been very profound. Other times the spoken words are, "I get it God THANK YOU." Even though many times the gift came out of a painful situation, I get it, God, I get it. Then my Spirit is filled with deep appreciation and gratitude.

~Phase 10~

Wisdom of the Spirit

I see through eyes of Spirit, and I am amazed at the resilience of life. I look around and see the ones who have shinned the light, on a path for others to walk. A path only you yourself can walk. Walk you will, with love on your side and peace in your heart. You will walk and the life you have lived will keep you moving forward. We are the children of the Divine. We are the Children of the Light. We have come here to this Beautiful Earth, to give God back his Creation. We are on the streets homeless, riding skateboards, and working in big corporations. We are all Nationalities and all different Faiths and Teachings, but we are One.

We are your Brother and Sisters, Daughters, and Sons. We are your Grandchildren, your Parents, and your Friends. We are your Wives, Husbands, and Partners.

We are the Demonstrators in the streets carrying signs of hope. We hope to bring the Darkness to the Light. We are the ones putting our Energy out there, from the Earth the Animals and all of Mankind. We believe the Earth and all life upon it is a gift from our Creator. Our journey is one in which, we may be the Stewards of this Earth, with honor and respect in our hearts, for this is loaned to us. It provides an opportunity to grow, so we can evolve Spiritually.

We are the ones that the Majority of people don't understand. We are the Energy of God that stands for change, stands for evolution of the Spirit. We feel it, and we believe in it. The brilliance of it all, we sense is an Honor that we can accept such a gift and in return, take care of it as God intended all of Creation to be cared for.

We are the Children of the Light. Sending that light out to all the Earth and the Universe that encompasses it. We came to bring the Light back to the Earth, in every form created. Light is our truth, love is our reminder of that truth. We are the Children of the Light because we let our light shine and honor the light in all of God's creation. Compassion shows us the way to embrace the Universal changes, which will awaken us to new life.

The awareness of life as energy vibrantly glowing and brilliantly healing speaks volumes to the enlightened voices being heard all over this beautiful planet that we call Mother Earth. **We take care of this Creation, for God has entrusted us to do so. We are the Children of the Light!!!**

The Wisdom of Spirit springs forth for all of us to explore and apply to our path. You can hear the Wisdom of Spirit in Nature, the Animals, and a child's laughter. You can see it with a smile, the Sunrise, and Sunset. The Wisdom of Spirit is all around us, just waiting for us to answer its call. It will speak to you however you listen.

In whatever way you perceive Spirit; it will speak to your Soul. Many will listen, but many will ignore it. Those who listen, give new life to Self and those they encounter. It is always a gentle nudging, a soft whisper beckoning us to remember our true self, our Spirit.

We are all the expressions of the Divine, waiting to be free, to express this light that shines so powerful in all of us. When we create an avenue for the light, it expands and flows in every direction we allow it.

The energy of the Spirit that inhabits the Human body is the true self of life. Think of your body as a container, a Temple of God's energy. A Temple, that shines. All the great Spiritual teachings throughout time, have taught that our bodies are a house or Temple for Spirit to express itself in, in this Earthly existence. God's energy is like a never-ending flowing current, always expanding and seeking new awareness. You are an ember of the Divine, waiting to shine. You speak the words of Spirit that most people only hear in their Soul. It is a soft whisper until its vibration becomes so loud that you can no longer ignore its force.

All around you the World you have come to know seems as if it is falling apart at its core. You know in your heart of hearts, this is not how this World was meant to express itself and all those who inhabit it.

We are all, the Children of the Light, and all are being called. Called to assist, in the liberation of a New Earth. Those who make the choice to Awaken within will share in a World that the Divine will be visible everywhere. What we choose in life now, will affect the beginning of the new life waiting to burst into existence.

"I See You"

I see you as the rain falls from the sky and dances to refresh Mother Earth.
I see you in the glowing Summer sky.

I felt you warm my body as the Sun released its heat upon the Earth. I see you through the eyes of the Deer as they pass on the trail beside me. I see you as the Hawk flies by.
I see you in the glimpse of the shadow that just passed me by.
I see you in the eyes of those around me.
I see you in the Mountain's River,
as it flows in harmony with the Heartbeat of Mother Earth.
I see you in the Ocean's waves as they flow in and out, with the rhythm of the Breath. "I see you, God I see you."
In all your creation, I see you.
"Know my child; it is I, who sees you. I Am the one who has been watching you! "
©2017

~PHASE 11~

Gateway's to my inner Consciousness turned Sanctuary within!

There have been so many gateways that have brought me back to my inner-self to Spirit, as far back as I can remember. Here are a few gateways that brought me back to my inner Sanctuary.

My Childhood, then my teen years. My sister's death was a huge gateway for growth, as was 29 years later catching the man who took my sister's life. As well as Breast Cancer, and Brain surgery to name a few. My mom's transition. The first book I had written "The Forgotten Temple" became a gateway.

There are so many gateways that can direct a person to go within. We are constantly being reminded of the Spirit within. To go inside ourselves and create an inner connection, to our Spirit where the Divine that resides within all of us, is a gift waiting to be opened and treasured. The Divine speaks to all. All who listen will find their way within, and create an inner awareness so beautiful and filled with such light, that it will flow out and be expressed in everyday life.

What creates your inner Sanctuary? We are all the Temples of the Divine. A Temple is a place of Worship, to honor the Divine within you. Your Temple can become a Sanctuary. The old ancient Spiritual teachings of Hindu, Buddhist, the Essenes, and many more old Spiritual teachings, all teach your body is a vessel, a Temple that houses your Soul.

A Sanctuary is a place of refugee, from the storms that you walk through in everyday life. Your Sanctuary should bring you peace. A peace so strong, that nothing can disturb its presence. Your Sanctuary should be a sacred place to your Soul, that the very act of everyday breathing is a safe and complacent part of your life. It is a place of unbending calm along with a sweet liberated love.

Your Sanctuary is of your own making. It is your energy that builds it strong, yet gentle as a way with the anticipation of serenity. The Mountains have always been a Sanctuary to me. They are strong and at the same time, Gentle. The Mountains breathe the Divine all over. When I leave the mountains, I take with me the energy that flows so freely through the trees, the calm and raging rivers, and the waterfalls. From the animals that live in the mountains to rocks and flowers all glowing with light, this energy fills my inner Sanctuary, my Temple.

The feeling of the cool breeze as it whispers past your ear, beckoning you to come play in God's Creation. All this energy that feeds your Soul is waiting to take its place in your inner Sanctuary.

You are the Temple of the Divine Energy; now turn your Temple into a Sanctuary of Peace and Safety.

Some of the Earth's Temples are in plain sight. The mountains are a Temple, as is the Ocean. The rivers and the trees they too are beautiful Temples. Nature is the playground of the Spirit. Nature sings the song of our Creator, reminding us of our true self within Spirit.

"All of my Life"

All of my life I felt and heard the call of Spirit guiding me, pushing me toward my true self.
I felt the Spirit's flow reaching a never-ending current of energy, as it moved through me.
The whisper never ended. I just did not always listen to it.

At times I brushed it off thinking little of it. At times it was so loud and it felt so strong I could not ignore it.

It is always here, Spirit is always here waiting for us!
©2000

~PHASE 12~

FREEDOM and GRATITUDE

Freedom comes in many different forms and from many different experiences. The freedom I am talking about came in the form of not having to take a medication that I had been on for 43 years. I was now free from having to take seizure medication along with freedom from seizures. The seizures are an experience in the past. I took a chance at a better life and now that chance has brought me full circle. It had been forty-three years, and now I was free to live life without seizures and the medication.

Having the freedom of not worrying about taking a drug anymore is compelling to itself. Frightening at first but oh so grateful as time went on. Freedom expresses itself in so many different forms.

The greatest feeling of freedom is to be free from the self-sabotaging thoughts of me, and the World around me. Free to express and believe in the life I partake in every day. Not all energy is going to flow with mine, but I can learn to allow it to flow by and not get stuck in it.

The freedom to express yourself and stand for what you believe in is a gift to all. Another Freedom is to believe and worship, as you express your devotion, to the light of God within you. God is freedom.

The freedom to express your awareness of a situation can bring growth to yourself, and others who can learn and grow from the sharing of life.

Freedom comes in many forms and expressions. One of my favorite sayings is "See how free you really are, check the hate in your heart".

Gratitude tells the Universe, "thank you, thank you for believing in me. My life is so blessed and I AM GRATEFUL FOR ALL THAT I AM AND ALL THAT IS IN MY LIFE." Gratitude is a gift from your heart back to God. An appreciation, of the life that you are. We take so much for granted.

Not even recognizing the gifts that are given to us every day. Some of those gifts are our eyesight. Watching the Sunrise, and set. To be a witness with the gift of sight, and see the beauty of the mountains, in all their glory. The Gratitude, of having the gift of hearing. The sounds of Nature are amazing. The Earth as her rivers flow and Oceans roar. The different sounds that music offers us. Along with the sound of laughter, to name just a few. So much more, if we just stop and breathe it all in.

"IT IS Time"

It is the beginning of a new and Awakened life. A New life, for all people to embrace and make whole.

We are one.

The timing is Gods and all mankind will be called.

Not all will listen, but all will be called.

We are one; we are all one and the same.

Let us begin again as we embrace our oneness.

We have to stop separating and stop segregating people from each other.

We all make up the Human Race, it is time we embrace oneness.

We are one!

©2018

"I look to you"

I look to you God and I see it's true.
We are one and the same, I was never lost with you.
I found you living inside me, dreaming, laughing and smiling.

You're alive inside me and you still dare to Dream beyond me.

I love you, God, it makes me smile that we are one and the same.

Of course, we are, I Am your child.

©2018

Your Toolbox

Meditation is one of the power tools of the Universe. Prayer and Forgiveness, all are power tools of the Universe you can place in your toolbox. This is the toolbox that you fill to get you through this journey of life. The toolbox, that is in your heart.

Non-judging, is an amazing tool to keep you from having to forgive. As life goes on you will continue to find the needed tools to carry with you throughout life. Mindfulness is an amazing tool.

Kindness, Gratitude, Compassion, and Patience are amazing tools. Laughter and a sense of Humor are tools that can bring you relief, in life and all its twists and turns. Whatever you find helps you through life put it in your toolbox and carry it with you.

Peace is a tool of exceptional energy. If you can hold on to Peace throughout your life, you will have a place of refuge to sink into.

What can you put in your toolbox to assist you through life? I carry my toolbox in my Heart, and my mind digs through it at very specific times, to assist my heart in staying open. Open, when it wants to close down, in this seemingly crazy World we are experiencing.

Keeping your heart open is an everyday task. You feed your reality every day with what you read, watch on television listen to on the radio. The different opinions of the people you surround yourself with. You are constantly feeding your reality. Keeping your heart open in the process is seemingly difficult at times. Be aware of what you are allowing into your everyday reality, it affects all areas of your life. It takes a good box of tools to navigate through life.

Worksheets

Make a List of Gateway's good or bad that has brought you to a new awakening in your life:

1.

2.

3.

4.

5.

6.

7.

List your closest friends and people you have meant along the way list what they did, that helped you through this Journey, called life:

1.

2.

3.

4.

5.

6.

7.

List the situations in your life that have brought you great healing, in Spirit, Mind, and Body:

1.

2.

3.

4.

5.

6.

7.

Now, list what you want to fill your inner consciousness/ Sanctuary with. List what can sustain you through the storms in life:

1.

2.

3.

4.

5.

6.

7.

List the areas of your life where you recognize your own Courage, and how you made it to the next day:

1.

2.

3.

4.

5.

6.

7.

**The End
of this story!**

www.ingramcontent.com/pod-product-compliance
Lightning Source LLC
Chambersburg PA
CBHW071411290426
44108CB00014B/1782